THE SCIENCE OF QUANTUM HEALING

Brian Glenn
&
Laura Shewfelt

innervisions
school of clinical hypnosis

CONTENTS

COPYRIGHT

DISCLAIMER

This book and its content do not provide medical advice and is not a substitute for medical advice or intervention.

The content is for informational purposes only.

Consult with your doctor (GP) on all medical issues regarding your condition and its treatment.

The content is not intended to be a substitute for professional medical advice, diagnosis, or treatment.

It is not a substitute for a medical examination, nor does it replace the need for services provided by a medical professional.

Always seek the advice of your medical professional before making any changes to your treatment. Any medical questions should be directed to your personal doctor.

Innervisions School of Clinical Hypnosis, or the book authors makes no warranties, either expressed or implied concerning the accuracy, applicability, reliability or suitability of the contents of this book.

Innervisions School of Clinical Hypnosis, or the book authors shall in no event be held liable for any direct, indirect incidental or other consequential damages arising directly or indirectly from any use of the information contained in this book.

All content is for information only and is not warranted for content accuracy or any other implied or explicit purpose.

ANCIENT WISDOM

The concept of energy fields has been present in many cultures and societies throughout history.

Our Ancient ancestors believed in the existence of unseen energies that permeated everything in the world, from people and animals to plants and rocks.

In ancient Chinese culture, the concept of "qi" (also known as chi or ki) was central to their understanding of the universe. It was believed that "qi" was the energy that flowed through all living things and that everything in the world was interconnected through this energy field.

Similarly, in Hindu culture, the concept of "prana" was central to their understanding of the universe. "Prana" was thought to be the life force energy that flowed through all living things and was responsible for maintaining balance and health in the body.

In Native American culture, the concept of the spirit world and the interconnectedness of all things was central to their beliefs. They believed that everything in the world had a spirit and that these spirits were connected through an energy field that permeated everything in the universe.

In ancient Egypt, the concept of “ma'at” was central to their understanding of the universe. “Ma'at” was the energy of balance and harmony that flowed through everything in the world, and it was believed that living in alignment with “ma'at” was essential for a person's spiritual and physical well-being.

Overall, the concept of energy fields has been a central part of many ancient cultures and remains an important part of spiritual and holistic practices today.

THE BEGINNING OF TIME

Let us start by going back to the beginning of time. Around the time 13 - 20 billion years ago, the universe as we knew it then was around the size of a green pea, and about 1cm in diameter.

This was probably because all the things we consider to be space in between everything, for example the space between us and the planet, the space between you and I, and the space between myself and this computer monitor was all considered to be non-existent.

Everything was compacted down to the size of a green pea, and because of this, the energy that was created was something around 1 million, million, degrees Fahrenheit. We are not really sure it was exactly one million, million, degrees Fahrenheit, we just know it was very, very, hot.

Then one day something magical happened. The energy that was generated in this matter actually exploded (the big bang) and that created the universe as we know it today. It created what we consider to have space between everything now.

So now there is space in-between the planets, space between you and me, space between you and this computer screen. Space if you look at it in a kind of a scientific way was created.

The picture on the left is of the neural network within the brain. The picture on the right was taken by the Hubble telescope and is a picture of the Universe.

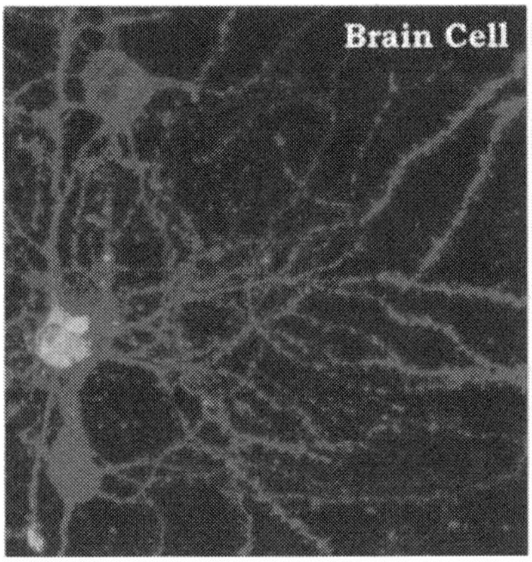

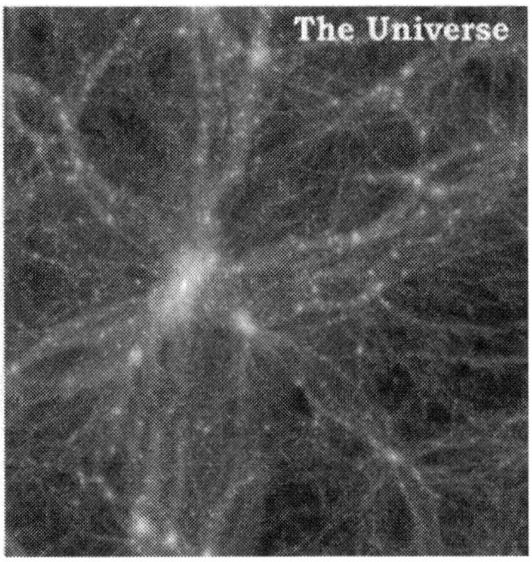

Notice the amazing similarities of the two pictures. This makes more sense of the passage seen in the bible

"As above – So below"

indicating that the biggest things we see in the universe are similar to the tiniest things in the universe.

ALBERT EINSTEIN

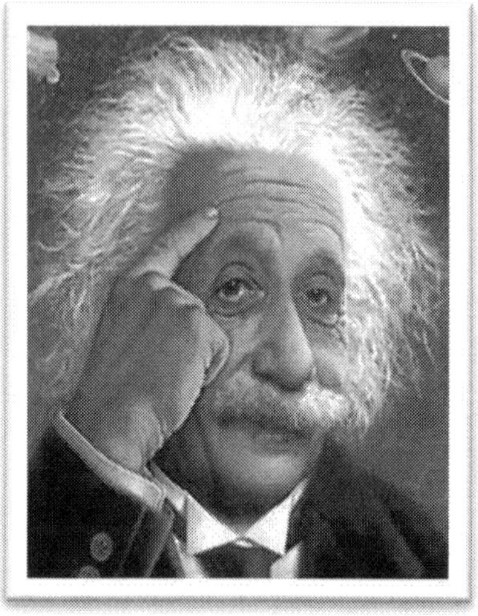

Albert Einstein had a bit of a problem with all this space and stuff; he claimed there couldn't be any space between us, and nothing in that space, he considered there must be something in that space. It is not empty space, so he declared.

He proposed there must be something in there, and he referred to this space as the Ether. He considered that if there was nothing there, then there wouldn't be any ability to shine light through anything, because there is nothing to shine the light through. There would be no ability to hear things because there would be nothing to transmit speech through. So, he considered there must be something in this empty space that he called the Ether.

Unfortunately, he could not prove the Ether existed, nor did he have the time to explore this, so what he decided to do was task a couple of his colleagues to conduct a scientific experiment to see if the Ether really did exist.

In the year 1897 – Einstein tasked two of his colleagues by the name of Michelson and Morley to come up with a scientific study to prove or disprove his theory that the Ether existed.

Michelson and Morley went ahead and built up a model to prove or disprove whether the Ether existed or not. They concluded by this scientific study that the Ether did not exist. This of course confused Einstein even more, he didn't like that at all, Einstein was adamant that the Ether did exist.

Over the next century it was considered that the Michelson and Morley experiment was the most famous failed experiment of all time because they discovered one hundred years later that the Ether does actually exist.

In 1986 a gentleman by the name of E. W. Silvertooth, who worked for the United States Air Force, repeated the experiment with more modern scientific equipment and he actually proved that the Ether does exist.

The Ether goes by lots of different names as it doesn't have an official name yet because it's still so young. Some people call it

- The Quantum Hologram
- Heaven
- The Field
- Natures Mind
- The Matrix

In more recent times there have been lots of experiments conducted to look at what is actually happening in this energy field.

An interesting experiment took place in Geneva on 25th July 1997 in the particle accelerator that exists there.

Imagine an underground tunnel that goes seven miles in one direction and seven miles in the other direction. What they did in Geneva was place a photon right in the middle as show in the diagram below.

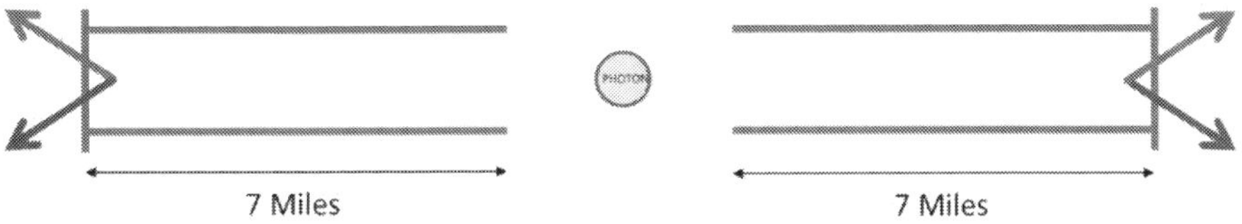

A photon of course is what everything is made up from. The photon was placed in the middle and then split into two and then the experiment began.

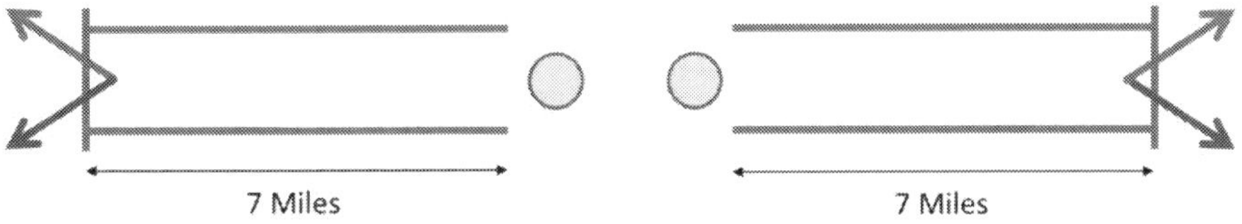

They fired each photon in the opposite directions all the way down to the end of the tube.

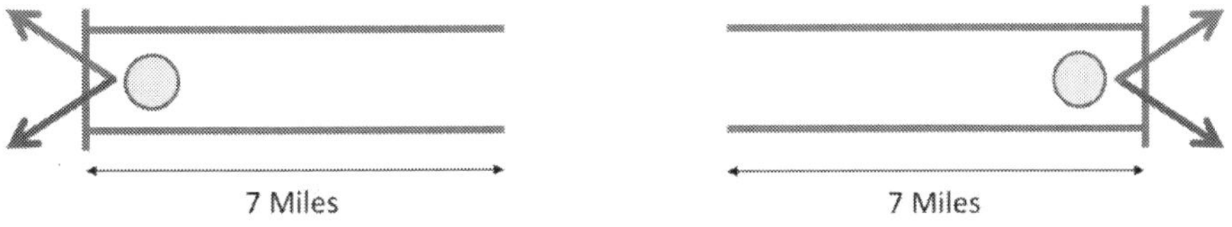

This in itself is not that difficult and not that unique, but what they found was when they took one of the photons, for example the one on the left and sent it up the green pathway, the right hand one also took the green pathway. And if they took the right hand one and sent it down the red pathway, the left one also went down the red pathway.

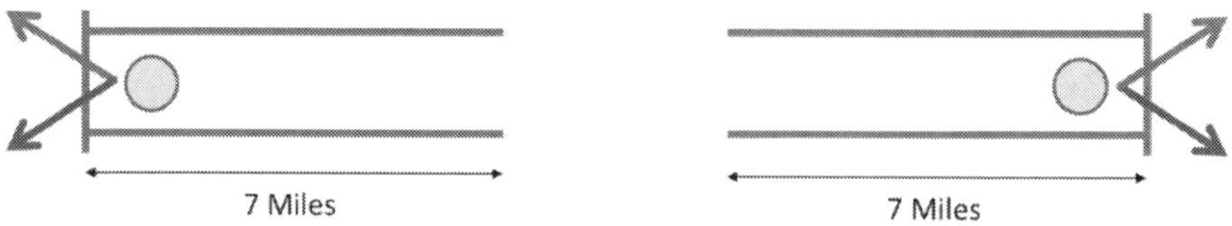

They considered this to be caused by the fact that the two photons were communicating with each other.

On further study they considered that the two photons could be communicating with each other, and if this was the case then there must be a time lapse between the communication. When looking at how long this time lapse was they realised there wasn't any and that it happened instantaneously.

For example if they sent the left hand photon up the green path, the right hand photon immediately went up the green path with no time lag, which proves without any doubt whatsoever that both photons are still connected together; a bit like when you see birds fly in the sky, when one turns, they all turn together, and with a shoal of fish when one turns, they all turn. This experiment concluded that we are still connected. After all, as human beings we are also made of photons; so, this proves we are all still connected, despite the big bang theory.

This theory was given a unique name - QUANTUM ENTANGLEMENT.

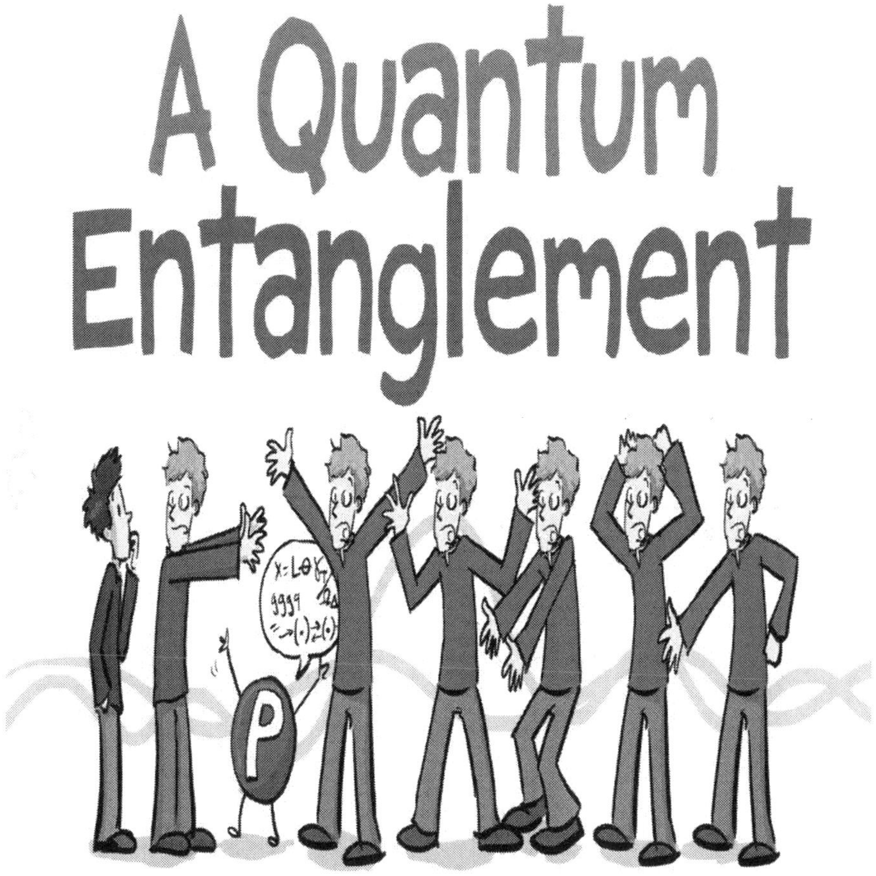

VISITING THE ENERGY FIELD

There is nothing really new here, but you may not have realised that us human beings visit the energy field on a regular basis.

For example:

- ✓ Natural sleep time
- ✓ Meditation
- ✓ Reiki
- ✓ Intimate sexual encounter
- ✓ Day dreaming
- ✓ During illness

NATURAL SLEEP:

It's pretty normal for most people to sleep on average 8 hours per day. So, if you live to be 90 you will have spent 30 years in the energy field. That's approximately one third of your life. Nature's way of natural healing. This is just one of the many reasons that it is important for us to maintain good sleep hygiene.

MEDITATION:

No wonder meditation is a viable healing modality. A way of quickly taking your body into the energy field for an energy boost.

REIKI:

According to the proven theory of quantum entanglement, it's pretty clear that reiki is a valid and worthy modality for healing. Sending symbols and healing thoughts through the energy field to help and heal the recipient.

INTIMATE SEXUAL ENCOUNTER:

Two lovers indulging in consenting intimate sex will always go into the energy field together, and later experience a massive feeling of peace and relaxation on their return to full consciousness. This is the place where new life comes from.

No wonder those who consciously try too hard to have a baby find it hard to conceive. Some even being told by medical 'experts' that they will never conceive, only to move on into a new, loving relationships and manifest a baby in this energy field.

Maybe this is why hypnosis for fertility is so successful. Many consider intimate sex to be a deep spiritual experience.

DAY DREAMING:

A brief and natural visit to the energy field to either focus on negative issues and inadvertently manifest negative realities, or focus on positive stuff and manifest the best future!

DURING ILLNESS:

When we are ill, we slip into the energy field often. Either by natural sleep or induced sleep and sometimes doctors will create a medically induced coma to allow your body to heal quicker. Children seem to sleep lots during illness, now we know why.

Animals also spend lots of time in the field. Perhaps they can actually see and sense the properties of the field. Sick animals heal there, they find comfort and safety there. When you see your dog 'apparently' sleeping on your sofa for many hours of the day, maybe your dog is NOT actually asleep, maybe they just go home for a bit ... to the energy field!

HYPNOTHERAPY IN THE ENERGY FIELD

For this to work at its best, you will now need to dump the scripts completely.

We now know, as fact, that we live in a diverse and infinite energy field which most animals can easily access on demand. Us human beings are also familiar with accessing this amazing energy field on a daily basis, particularly during our cycles of sleep although you may not realise it.

We can indeed make massive changes in our own life during the periods of our sleep cycle called the Hypnagogic and Hypnopompic state. More on this later.

First, let's examine the way in which we communicate with this energy field with all its infinite possibilities.

The energy field does not understand our verbal language, no matter what nationality we are. Instead, it understands the language that all nationalities understand; that of icons processed by our imagination. This applies to all animals too, they communicate with the very same energy field using icons and symbols.

So, we communicate with icons and emotion.

It is also our belief, that due to the fact that this energy field contains all the knowledge that ever existed, as well as all knowledge that the future holds in infinite time, that psychics and mediums are probably unwittingly accessing the very same energy field. Using it to retrieve data regarding their clients, as well as information regarding deceased loved ones.

The psychic actually goes into a trance like state and goes into the energy field. Wow, could this be scientific evidence that psychics have a real verified skill?

Brian stumbled upon this ability to literally connect to other people whilst in the hypnotic state many years ago, but he never fully understood how it actually worked and the power of instinct and intuition always seemed a bit ‘spooky’. But now we know more about this evidence-based energy field, we can attribute that to his ignorance from the past.

When we work with a client, and relax, and allow ourselves to drift into the energy field, we both meet there. Although we could actually be thousands of miles apart we almost become at one with our client and instinctively know what to say and how to say it.

One of the rules is that we must never hold anything back, whatever you say must not be censored in any way as the information is actually coming from source. Use language patterns that allow your client to create emotions and icons (visualisation).

PHYSICAL ILLNESS

From a perspective of physical illness, we can utilise the infinite possibilities of this field and actually take our client back to source, and return to the conscious state with miraculous changes having taken place in the physiological state of our client (or ourselves). Real physical healing of many life-threatening diseases can take place. Some of which have been deemed by medics as being terminal or chronic illnesses and conditions.

CELLULAR MEMORY

Taking another brief trip to Brian's early days as a hypnotherapist, he was always amazed by our bodies ability to reproduce cells every single day. Some cells taking days and other weeks months or years. But every time those brand-new body cells renewed themselves, the cells were reproduced identically to the last one. So, for example, if you have a scar on your leg, the scar will renew regularly and it will reproduce the same identical scar. Even though the scar was caused from an injury sustained many years ago, the body is actually producing a brand spanking new scar.

So, think about it. The legs you have today are not the same legs that you had this time last year, but they have identical characteristics. What if we could get our cells to grow without these characteristics? To make brand a new leg with no scars. Or a brand-new lung with no cancer (it's probably not even the same cancer that initially grew all those months ago anyway!).

Cellular memory is also responsible for the ageing process. As we grow old and the skin cells around our face get damaged from various life occurrences, pollution etc., so the body gets rid of the damaged cells (a natural process called "Apopstosis").

It then reproduces new cells that are identical to the last one, thus creating a chain of destruction (ageing).

Imagine if we could stop this cellular memory process at our prime age and maintain our exterior beauty!

All of this makes so much sense and accounts for many spontaneous recoveries from terminal illness, psychic readings, psychic predictions, the placebo effect, the nocebo effect, and it could even answer the long debate regarding what happens to us after death. Perhaps we simply return to where we came from in the first place, the energy field.

At this time, we have no way of scientifically validating the above, nor do we have the resources and finances to scientifically research this, but it won't be long before someone does!

In my younger years I used to wonder why it was that ill people heal better while they are sleeping. Even doctors put seriously ill people into coma states in order for the body to heal. Most elderly and terminally ill people actually die during sleep when their time on this earthly plain has ended.

It's all pretty obvious now, because when we sleep, we actually go into the energy field so that our bodies can heal. This is why it's so important to ensure that your sleep habits and patterns are good!

DELIVERING YOUR THERAPY IN THE FIELD

Keep it simple as always.

Just a normal unscripted basic induction,
Followed by a deepener of choice.

Close your eyes during this time and go with your own words too. (You can always open your eyes to observe any head nods if needed).

Then when the time is right, your own subconscious will have full access to all the knowledge and techniques you learned from your tutor (it's all there in this energy field). Let what you need come to you naturally and easily.

At first, you might feel like you are just randomly waffling away, but everything you say will actually be meaningful to your client. Don't force anything, just relax and go with the flow. If you can't think of anything to say, it's perfectly OK, simply keep quiet until you do have something to say.

Again, you can't do this using a script, reading a script is a conscious function.

If you are using one of the procedures where you need to write things down, Submodalities for example, just remain calm and relaxed (still in hypnosis) and begin to write stuff down. Remember that neither of you need to keep your eyes closed to remain in hypnosis (in the energy field).

The more you practice this, the better you will become at it and it won't be long till you have razor sharp instincts and intuition which you can easily access on demand.

WORKING IN THE HYPNAGOGIG AND HYPNOPOMPIC STATE

This section is all about YOU.

Here we present a unique and almost guaranteed way to resolve everyday issues, find answers, and find solutions to almost everything.

I (Brian) actually wrote most of the course material in the hypnagogic state and more recently discovered solutions for issues which arose whilst installing a new kitchen. It really is limitless and endless and an absolute must for personal development. You'll find the answers to everything there!

You may recall from Module One that there are two hypnosis states which all humans experience daily.

- The hypnagogic state
- The hypnopompic state

Unlike REM dreams which take place later on in the sleep cycle and often tend to follow a narrative, hypnagogic and hypnopompic dreams consist more of random, disassociated thoughts.

Hypnagogia is often accompanied by strange imagery, sounds and sensations. Many people experience visual hallucinations during hypnagogia. Most commonly these take the form of an elaborate, abstract visual interplay of light and geometry, sometimes interspersed with more recognisable images and forms.

Some people also experience auditory hallucinations; random sounds, speech or even musical fragments. Another example is the so-called Tetris Effect, whereby repetitive activities from your waking life permeate into your hypnagogic imagery.

As well as anecdotal evidence, scientific research also suggests that hypnagogic dreams are useful in solving problems that require creative insight.

In addition to the sensory curiosities of hypnagogic and hypnopompic dreams, there are some very interesting cognitive processes occurring.

Throughout history, visions, prophesies, premonitions and apparitions have all been the likely result of hypnagogic phenomena.

Researchers have described hypnagogia as involving a 'loosening of ego boundaries, openness, sensitivity, 'heightened suggestibility', and a 'fluid association of ideas'.

In layman's terms, this state is associated with more random associations of ideas than is normal, resulting in a state of heightened creativity.

FAMOUSLY HYPNAGOGIC

For a long time, Hypnagogia has been a gateway to creativity and productivity. Thomas Edison and Salvador Dali were two of the most notable people that made practical use of this free-thinking mindset.

Edison was an extremely motivated inventor and claimed that sleep was a waste of time, merely a remnant of our caveman days. This led him to develop some interesting sleep habits and it is well known that he was a big fan of naps.

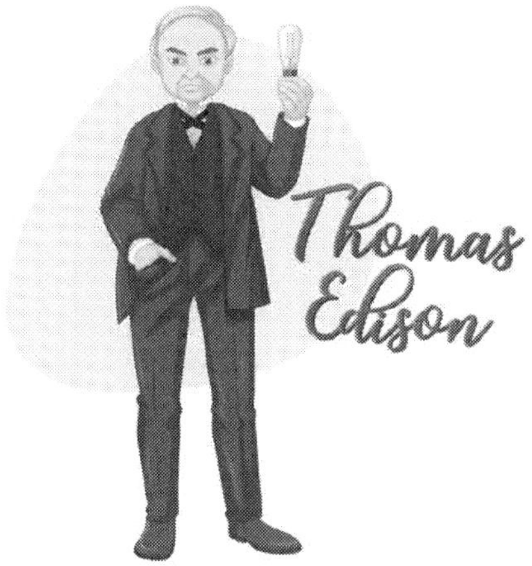

Less well known is Edison's hypnagogic habit. Holding a handful of steel ball bearings, he would settle into one of his famous naps. As soon as his hand relaxed, he would drop the ball bearings, waking him up in time to jot down his thoughts.

Salvador Dali used a similar technique. Rather than ball bearings, Dali would rest in his favourite chair, dangling a large key pinched between his thumb and forefinger above a plate sitting on floor. As unconsciousness swept over him, he would drop the key onto the plate and the resulting noise would snap him back to waking consciousness.

How to harness your hypnagogic potential

If you are interested in experimenting with the power of hypnagogic and hypnopompic dreams, I've devised a few techniques to maximize the benefits from mini naps and the hypnagogic state. The basic steps are as follows.

Incubate your ideas:

Saturating your brain with information related to the subject that you wish to dream/think about before laying down for a nap will increase the likelihood that your dreams will be related to that subject.

Get the timing right:

In order to benefit from your hypnagogic dreams, you need to time your naps correctly. If you're too sleepy when you lie down, you might fall into a deeper sleep or ignore your cue to get up.

Use a dreamcatcher:

Whether you go for a low-tech solution like Edison's ball-bearings or something more modern like my electronic dream catcher, you'll need a device to startle you into wakefulness at the opportune time.

Take notes immediately:

It's likely that any inspiration you gather from the hypnagogic state will fade pretty quickly. So, you should have a pen and notebook, or voice recorder right by your side, before your ideas disappear.

Today, we share with you these new ideas, perhaps attaining the 'Holy Grail' of healing, or at least being party to that goal.

Just as the energy field is a source of infinite knowledge and infinite possibilities, you now have similar infinite knowledge and wisdom to bring out the very best version of you.

Never be afraid to step out of that comfort zone and explore new ideas and techniques.

QUANTUM HEALING

Quantum healing uses the principles of quantum physics to promote healing and balance in the body.

It is based on the principle that everything in the universe is interconnected, and that energy is at the core of all matter. We are of course all made up of energy.

As you know everything in the universe is made up of energy, and that energy is constantly vibrating at different frequencies. When the energy in the body is out of balance or blocked, it can lead to physical and emotional health problems.

Many Quantum healers believe that by manipulating the energy fields around the body, they can promote healing and restore balance to the body. They use methods such as reiki, visualisation and meditation.

We believe that hypnosis and hypnotherapy is an even more powerful technique to rebalance and restore and heal the body from the inside. Using the hypnotized subjects own mind and body system to bring health and healing.

Brian has pioneered a method of doing this and will demonstrate it at the live event.

Let's look at the 12 Universal Laws under which we all operate under and are subject to.

These reinforce this theory of interconnectedness and that the key to health and wellness lies in this energy field of which we all are part of.

THE 12 UNIVERSAL LAWS

The 12 Universal Laws are irrefutable explanations of how things operate in this time-space reality. These laws weren't created by mankind and now can they be destroyed.

They simply describe how things ARE.

The 12 universal laws originated from Source - also known as God, the Universe, The Matrix, Higher Power, or the Energy Field as we prefer to call it.

Just like physical laws such as the Law of Gravity, these Universal Laws were not invented but in fact have been discovered by humans through our observations and experiences.

The Law of Gravitation existed way before it was discovered by Isaac Newton and there are probably many other Universal Laws for us to still discover!

The 12 Laws of the universe describe the way things operate in this universe and because they are always working, whether you are aware of them or not, understanding them puts you at an advantage in life. And vice versa of course!

They are like the rules of the game, so to speak. If you want to win the game, you must first learn the rules or in this case the Laws!

Understanding the Laws of the Universe can help you to not only survive but thrive in the universe.

At present there is a total of 12 Laws of the Universe that are widely accepted to be true. There are probably many other laws in play at any given moment, however, not every law has been discovered or given a name yet.

The main one is the ***Law of Divine Oneness***.

This fundamental Law states that everything is connected and nothing is truly separate from each other.

This Law helps you to remember that no matter what happens in this physical reality, you are never separated from source or from each other on a spiritual level.

The Law of Divine Oneness can bring inner peace and relief to any earthly problems because you can stay grounded in the knowledge that all is well on the spiritual level, which is the truth of who you are.

Let's look at them in order:

1. The Law of Divine Oneness

As discussed previously, the Law of Divine Oneness is the first of the 12 Universal Laws.

It helps us to understand that everything is connected to everything else and it is the foundational Law of the Universe.

All our thoughts, words, actions and beliefs affect us, others, and the universe around us. This is irrespective of whether others are near or far away, in other words, we are all connected beyond time and space.

Everything in the Universe is an extension of Source energy which means nothing is separate on a spiritual level.

You practice this law when you exercise compassion and consciously recognize that ultimately we are all one being. As hypnotherapists this is a gift to us as we can connect with our clients as one during the session.

2. The Law of Vibration

The Law of Vibration states that everything in the Universe vibrates, moves, and travels in circular patterns. Whether tangible or intangible, everything is made up of energy that is vibrating at a specific frequency.

The same principle of vibration in the physical world applies to our internal world in terms of our feelings, desires, thoughts.

Everything that you see, like your phone, your pets, your friends, and everything that you don't see, such as your thoughts, feelings, and emotions, is comprised of energy that is constantly vibrating.

Each sound, thought or thing has its own unique vibrational frequency. When you hear people say 'like attracts like', they are actually referring to how a vibrational energy can resonate with or is attracted to the same or a similar vibrational energy.

This is the reason why what others do or say affects us directly or indirectly. If you are not happy with your current vibration, you need to make a conscious choice to focus your energy more on positive emotions. This will raise your vibration higher. Also, by giving others that which you desire, you indirectly increase that which comes back to you.

Of course, when you pair the Law of Vibration with the Law of Attraction, you have the formula of what it takes to attract your desires into your reality through vibrational alignment.

To manifest your desires using the Law of Vibration, all you have to do is identify the vibration of your desire and then raise your vibration until you become a vibrational match with what you want.

By the Law of Attraction, your vibration will attract things, people, situations, experiences, and outcomes with the same vibration into your life.

3. The Law of Inspired Action

The Law of Inspired Action states that inspiration will come about when you are aligned with who you are;

an extension of Source as stated by the Law of Divine Oneness.

The Law of Inspired Action must be applied in order for us to create things, therefore, we must engage in actions that support our words, feelings, vision, thoughts, dreams and emotions. These actions will bring us manifestations that a match to our specifically chosen words, thoughts, dreams, and emotions.

Practicing this Law is all about slowing down, getting quiet, and creating space for guidance to come forward. When we let go of our need to control how things will work out and are instead open to all possibilities, it makes room for new ways of achieving the goals that we might not have considered otherwise.

4. The Law of Correspondence

The Law of Correspondence puts us in the drivers' seat of our own lives.

Our outer world is a direct reflection of our inner world, therefore, we need to accept responsibility for our own lives.

Our current reality is a mirror of what is going on inside of us. A result of our innermost dominant though:

"As within, so without"

"As above, so below"

The Law of Correspondence states that your external reality is a direct reflection of your internal state. This law makes it pretty easy to assess the alignment of your vibration.

If your life is chaotic and out of order, not serving you then it means your vibration is out of alignment. However, if your life appears to be thriving, it means your vibration is in alignment.

5. The Law of Cause and Effect

The Law of Cause and Effect, states that ***nothing*** happens by chance or outside the Universal Laws.

This means that, we must take responsibility for everything that happens in our lives. Every action has a reaction or consequence and what we sow is what we reap.

The Law of Cause and Effect, states that for every cause there's an effect.

In life, our thinking is the cause and our experiences are the effects of our thinking.

Trying to change our experiences without looking at the cause is a 'sticking plaster' solution, because all negative experiences are merely the effects of our thinking.

So, if you want to change your experience, you must begin by changing your thoughts.

6. The Law of Compensation

This Law of Compensation is the extended arm of the Law of Cause and Effect which is applied to abundance and good things that flow into our lives in the form of friendships, gifts, money, inheritances etc. These various forms of compensation are the visible effects of our direct and indirect actions carried out throughout our lives.

The Law of Compensation states that you reap what you sow.

What you give to others shall be given to you.

What you withhold from others shall be withheld from you.

If you offer your highest and best to everyone and everything in life, you will be rewarded with the highest and best.

7. The Law of Attraction

This Law of Attraction shows how we create the events, people and things that come into our lives. All our thoughts, words, feelings and actions give out energies which, likewise attract like energies.

Positive energies will always attract positive energies while negative energies will always attract negative energies. It doesn't matter whether you want the negative or not. What you place your attention on, is what you attract into your life.

The Law of Attraction states "that which is like onto itself is drawn".

This law applies to everything that exists in the universe from tangible things like objects, people, and situations to intangible things like thoughts, feelings, and emotions.

This is why people experience phenomena like a lucky streak or a downward spiral.

It is no coincidence that when things get good, it gets better. And when things get worse, it gets way worse. It's simply the Law of Attraction in action.

Of course, ultimately it all comes down to your energy. Your energy is constantly attracting situations, events, and experiences that are a direct match to it.

By applying the Law of Attraction to your own life, you will have absolute clarity over why situations occur the way they do and more importantly, what you can do to shift your energy and change the outcomes you receive.

8. The Law of Perpetual Transmutation of Energy

The Law of Perpetual Transmutation of Energy is a powerful one.

It states that we all have power within us to change any condition in our lives that we are not happy with.

Higher energy vibrations will definitely consume and transform lower ones. Because the Law of Perpetual Transmutation of Energy states that energy is constantly evolving or fluctuating, we can change the energies in our lives.

This law makes perfect sense because the Law of Vibration states that everything is energy and the Law of Attraction states that like attracts like.

Your energy is always moving towards high vibration (positivity) or low vibration (negativity). So, it is your job to monitor your vibration alignment and direct your focus towards better-feeling thoughts when necessary.

9. The Law of Relativity

The Law of Relativity states that each person will receive a series of situations or problems for the purpose of strengthening us.

We should consider each of these tests to be a challenge and remain connected to our hearts when solving the problems.

This law also teaches us to compare our situations to other people's problems and put everything into its right perspective. No matter how bad we perceive our situations to be, there is always someone who is in a more difficult or worst situation, thereby making it all relative.

The Law of Relativity states that everything is relative because we all perceive reality in our own way.

This Law explains why two people can go through the same situation but have two entirely different experiences and responses.

Understanding this Law helps you prioritise inner peace over defending the truth because “truth” is relative anyway.

10. The Law of Polarity

The Law of Polarity states that everything is on a continuum and has an opposite. There has to be darkness so that we might appreciate Light. There is solid and liquid and we can see and feel the difference. We have the ability to suppress and transform undesirable thoughts by focusing on the opposite thought thereby bringing the desired positive change.

The Law of Polarity states that everything in life has an opposite.

For every problem, there's a solution. For every obstacle, there's an opportunity.

This Law is what gives birth to new desires when manifesting.

Every time you experience something you don't want, this law points out that the thing you do want exists and is just waiting to be manifested into your life.

11. The Law of Rhythm

The Law of Rhythm states that everything vibrates and moves to a certain rhythm.

This rhythm establishes cycles, seasons, patterns, and stages of development. Each cycle is a reflection of the regularity of the universe. To master each rhythm, you must rise above any negative part of the cycle.

The Law of Rhythm states that cycles are a natural part of the Universe. Just like the four seasons, your life has seasons too.

Surrender to the flow of life and let your inner wisdom guide your thoughts, words, and actions.

12. The Law of Gender

The Law of Gender states that everything has masculine (yang) and feminine (yin) principles, and that these are the basis for all creation in the Universe. As spiritual beings, we must balance between the masculine and feminine energies within us in order for us to become true co-creators.

The Law of Gender states that life works best when your divine masculine and divine feminine energies are in alignment.

The divine feminine represents the part of our consciousness that connects us to qualities like intuition, feeling, emotions, creativity, and spirituality.

This feminine energy is the exact opposite of the divine masculine which connects us to qualities like logic, authority, confidence, objectivity, and action-taking.

One thing to note is that one is not better than the other. Both the divine feminine and the divine masculine need to work together harmoniously to create solutions for the highest good.

However, society has traditionally favoured masculine qualities over feminine qualities. This is why we must restore our connection to our divine feminine to restore balance in our lives.

YOUR PERSONAL FREQUENCY

In essence, nothing would exist without thoughts and vibrations.

We influence our reality every second based on our thoughts and vibrations. In other words, we create our reality according to the frequency at which we are operating.

By increasing your frequency, you will have a much easier time attracting things and people into your existence, which you want and that positively affect you. You will also ensure that all the cells in your body are vibrating at a frequency of health.

"If you want to find the secrets of the universe, think in terms of energy, frequency and vibration."
Nikola Tesla

We all have a personal vibration that radiates from us and it changes depending on what we're thinking, feeling, and doing.

"You can let your personal vibration match the world's chaotic soup of frequencies and feel buffeted about helplessly, or you can determine how you want to feel...Your personal vibration or energy state is a blend of the contracted or expanded frequencies of your body, emotions, and thoughts at any given moment. The more you allow your soul to shine through you, the higher your personal vibration will be."

Penney Peirce, Frequency: The Power of Personal Vibration

We're not only affected by our own vibrations but also from the vibrations of everything around us - from people, places, and things. Since everything is energy and we are connected, it makes sense that all vibrations have an effect on us both positively or negatively.

The good news is that we can decide the frequency we want to live in because we have the power to influence our own personal vibration.

Your life expands when you're living in a higher vibrational frequency.

When you move up the ladder vibrationally it affects your reality and your life begins to flow in many different areas, from your relationships and health to your career and finances.

Not only is your life more harmonious, but as Wayne Dyer writes in his book "Intention":

"The higher your energy, the more capable you are of nullifying
and converting lower energies, which weaken you."

Dr. David R. Hawkins, the author of Power vs. Force, created a "Map of Consciousness" which actually depicts the different energy fields of consciousness and the vibrational levels in which we live.

Our consciousness levels are determined by our emotions, perceptions, attitudes, world views and spiritual beliefs. The map ranges from 20 - 1000 and he says that the collective level of consciousness is currently at 207.

The critical response point in the scale of consciousness calibrates at level 200, which is the level associated with integrity and courage.

All attitudes, thoughts, feelings, associations below that level of calibration make a person go weak; those that calibrate higher make subjects go strong. This is the balance point between weak and strong attractors, between negative and positive influence.

Dr. David R. Hawkins -

Those that are living below the level of 200 are mainly in survival mode and are destructive of life. As a person passes the 200 level, which is between the negative and positive energies, they move into courage and the well-being of others.

- At the 500 level: Both the happiness and spiritual awareness for oneself and others is important.

- By the 600's: You're dealing with the good of mankind and search for enlightenment.

- From 700 to 1,000: Life is dedicated to the salvation of humanity - it's here that you find the enlightened ones: Buddha, Jesus Christ, and Krishna.

Map of Consciousness

Developed By David R. Hawkins

	Name of Level	Energetic Log	Predominant Emotional State	View of Life	God-view	Process
Spiritual Paradigm	Enlightenment	700-1000	Ineffable	Is	Self	Pure Consciousness
	Peace	600	Bliss	Perfect	All-Being	Illumination
	Joy	540	Serenity	Complete	One	Transfiguration
	Love	500	Reverence	Benign	Loving	Revelation
Reason & Integrity	Reason	400	Understanding	Meaningful	Wise	Abstraction
	Acceptance	350	Forgiveness	Harmonious	Merciful	Transcendence
	Willingness	310	Optimism	Hopeful	Inspiring	Intention
	Neutrality	250	Trust	Satisfactory	Enabling	Release
	Courage	200	Affirmation	Feasible	Permitting	Empowerment
Survival Paradigm	Pride	175	Scorn	Demanding	Indifferent	Inflation
	Anger	150	Hate	Antagonistic	Vengeful	Aggression
	Desire	125	Craving	Disappointing	Denying	Enslavement
	Fear	100	Anxiety	Frightening	Punitive	Withdrawal
	Grief	75	Regret	Tragic	Disdainful	Despondency
	Apathy	50	Despair	Hopeless	Condemning	Abdication
	Guilt	30	Blame	Evil	Vindictive	Destruction
	Shame	20	Humiliation	Miserable	Despising	Elimination

SOME EASY WAYS TO RAISE YOUR OWN FREQUENCY

1. Eat Natural Foods

Dense foods such as meats, processed foods, and alcohol lower your vibration. Eating foods that don't come from nature weigh you down and therefore decrease your frequency. However, eating lighter meals that have a lower karmic load, such as fruits and veggies, will naturally raise your energy levels. Foods that come from nature have life force energy.
Boxed foods and meats have much less life force energy, making you feel dull and unenthusiastic about life. If you want to feel more vibrant, here are some foods to include in your diet:

- fruits
- veggies
- nuts
- seeds
- grains
- raw dairy
- eggs

Avoid alcohol and any mind-altering substances as well, they act as depressants that numb you, which will negatively impact you in the long run.

2. Be mindful of what your mind consumes.

Just as the foods we eat can either increase or decrease our vibration, so can the types of entertainment we allow into our lives.

Overconsumption of news and social media can literally drain our life force energy. Much of the media focuses on the negative occurrences in our world, so watching too much of it will raise cortisol levels and cause fear.

The entertainment we choose should uplift us and give us a sense of peace and happiness. Anything that causes discord or fear in our energy field should either be eliminated or significantly reduced to uplift our energy.

Instead of spending hours scrolling social media, which tends to leave people feeling anxious and depressed, why not watch an inspirational video or funny TV show? What we give our attention to expands in our consciousness, and by feeding our brains positive information, our whole world will start to become brighter and our personal frequency instantly responds.

3. Get out into nature!

One of the best ways to raise your frequency is right outside your front door!

We evolved to spend plenty of time in the sunshine, but our modern environments filled with overstimulation and artificial lighting have far removed us from what our bodies need.

Make sure you spend at least 15-30 minutes per day getting some fresh air, and sunlight. Vitamin D can help alleviate depression and boost your immune system.

Feel the earth directly underneath your feet and its natural vibration. The earth's vibration is healing, rejuvenating, balancing and uplifting.

4. Practice meditation, breathing exercises, self-hypnosis and heart coherency.

Focus on deep breathing and go deep within to access inner self. All of these offer great opportunities to increase your frequency while also providing many health benefits, such as better concentration, lower stress, reduced blood pressure and heart disease, among others.

Quieten the mind and pay attention to the breath, will ground you in the present moment. Eventually, you'll notice racing thoughts will start to dissipate, and you'll have much less attachment to them. Many people allow their thoughts to torment them, but in these states, you realise that you exist beyond your mind.

5. Move your body.

Raising your frequency mostly involves taking care of your mind and body properly. In our fast-paced world, many of us neglect our mental and physical health, which only lowers our vibration.

Not only does exercise improve our physical health, but it keeps our minds healthy as well. Choose whatever kind of exercise makes you feel good.

6. Focus on gratitude, love, appreciation and generosity.

Our emotions play a major role in determining our frequency. High vibe emotions like love and appreciation make us feel lighter and more vibrant, while negative feelings like anger and envy cause heaviness within the body.

This doesn't mean you shouldn't listen to your feelings, just don't allow yourself negative ones to take you over. Allow them to pass through you, take what you need from the message they are giving you and then turn your focus to taking action and to higher vibrational emotions.

7. Fill your inner circle with positive people.

Don't allow people to steal your energy away, make sure you surround yourself with an inner circle of positive people who will uplift you.

Negative people tend to drain others of power because they have none to offer themselves, so avoid these types of energy vampires whenever possible.

You will probably attract them because of your infectious positivity, but limit your exposure!

HEART AND BRAIN COHERENCE

Heart and brain coherence is the unity and integration of mind, body, and spirit. It is when our thoughts, intentions, and actions seamlessly align. It not only has powerful effects on our mental and emotional health, stability and resilience but also on our physical health. It can affect heart rate, immune system, sleep quality, and overall energy levels.

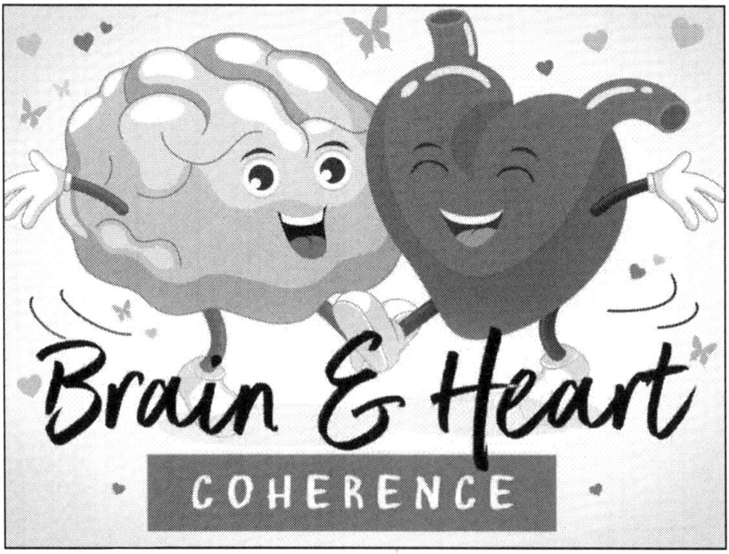

When there is a strong heart and brain connection, then we are able to think more clearly, focus better, and experience heightened emotional well-being. Let's look at some of the benefits of living in a state of heart and mind coherence from mental, emotional, and physical perspectives because they are vast.

1. Feeling Whole

Brain and heart coherence entails unconditional acceptance of what is, so when we practice it, we exist in the now, as opposed to living in the future or dwelling on the past. This helps us feel whole without the need to escape anything.

2. Feeling Unity with Yourself and the World

The more we accept ourselves and our life the way it is, the deeper our sense of unity with ourselves and the world becomes. We breathe life in freely, without fighting anything, and that fosters deep relaxation and the feeling of being in harmony with the world.

3. Deep Inner Peace

The more heart-centered actions we take, the more we teach our minds to believe that no matter what happens, we will always have our own backs and we will always be okay. With this comes deep trust in ourselves and our personal power, which brings about feelings of deep inner peace.

4. Decreased Stress

When we fully accept our life the way it is, breathe it in, and allow our bodies to experience it, the less we feel the need to worry about the future or dwell in the past. With acceptance comes letting go and far less to stress about. Because once again, when we take actions that serve our hearts, our mind learns that no matter what happens, we will be okay. As we have now become our own protectors, our own best friends, and our own partners in crime.

5. Increased Energy & Vitality

When we are in a state of coherence, we think less and feel way more. Moreover, with aligned actions, there is suddenly no need to dwell. Heart speaks very clearly and gives obvious directions. When we align our efforts with the heart's desires and act from there, so much energy is saved because we are not constantly worrying and ruminating anymore. We have a clear destination and can use all our energy toward the action.

6. Enhanced Creativity

The less we think, the more space we have in our minds. And the more we feel, the more we tap into the flow of our creative energy. Suddenly, we start getting more creative ideas about situations in our life that we would have never thought of before, more ideas about how to creatively express who we are. And when we take action on these ideas, the joy generated by our decisions creates palpable ripples in all areas of our lives.

7. Emotional Intelligence and Mastery

When we align the mind, body, and soul, we stop running from our emotions and start running toward them. We willingly jump into the sea of our deep emotional hearts because we are not afraid anymore. Instead, we:

- ✓ Start acknowledging them all as our own
- ✓ Start understanding where they come from and why
- ✓ Start taking full responsibility for them
- ✓ Start channelling them on our life's purpose

8. Greater Resilience

When we teach our brain that no matter what, we will always have our own back, we become incredibly resilient. When challenging situations try to knock the breath out of us, we know how to act. We feel all there is to handle, and then we take a deep breath and keep moving.

9. Solid Mental Health

Solid mental health lies in trust. Living in a coherent state requires a deeply trusting relationship you're your heart. Once that trust is established, there is a solid foundation that no one but you can ruin. No outside circumstances could erode this trust, as it is built on actions you choose to take.

10. Improved Physical Health

Research shows that the state of coherence improves your immune function, decreases stress hormones, improves heart health, and promotes overall wellness. This is the true "health inside-out" phenomenon that could be easily achieved and measured.

11. Deeper Emotional Connection with Yourself and Others

The deeper you dive into your own emotions and the more compassion you feel for yourself, the deeper you will be able to dive with others, creating incredible relationships rooted in honesty and authenticity.

12. Improved Quality of Life Overall

Life becomes lighter, more prosperous, deeper, joyful, and meaningful. The more of this richness you have, the more you want, naturally creating more joy, energy, and vitality.

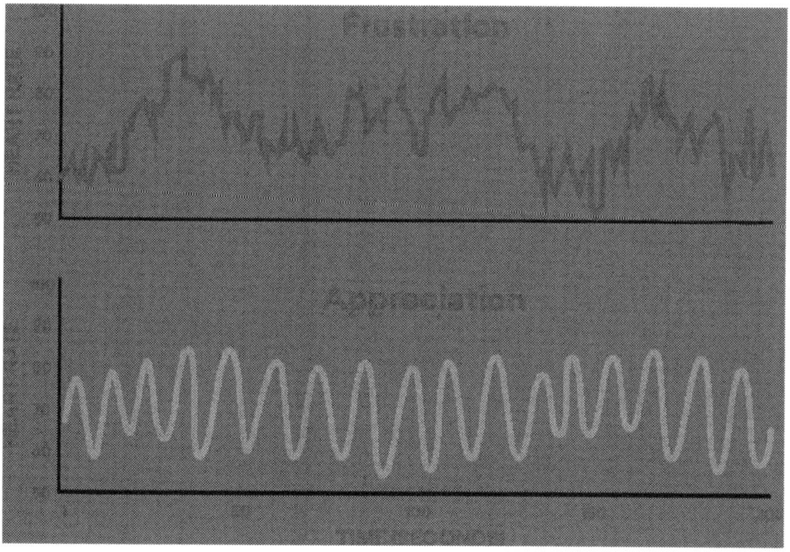

THE SCHUMANN RESONANCE

The Schumann resonance is often referred to as the heartbeat of Mother Earth or the earth's vibration and is actually a frequency.

It's the measurement of 7.83 Hz or the electromagnetic frequency of our planet, to be exact.

The Schumann Resonance is said to not only affect the earth, but also align or implement changes in human consciousness.

This energy can increase or decrease at times, and many think it affects our consciousness. Is this true? Well, let's take a look at the facts we know first.

It starts with electrical storms. These are more than just spectacles and frightening events. An electrical storm generates lightning, which creates electromagnetic energy.

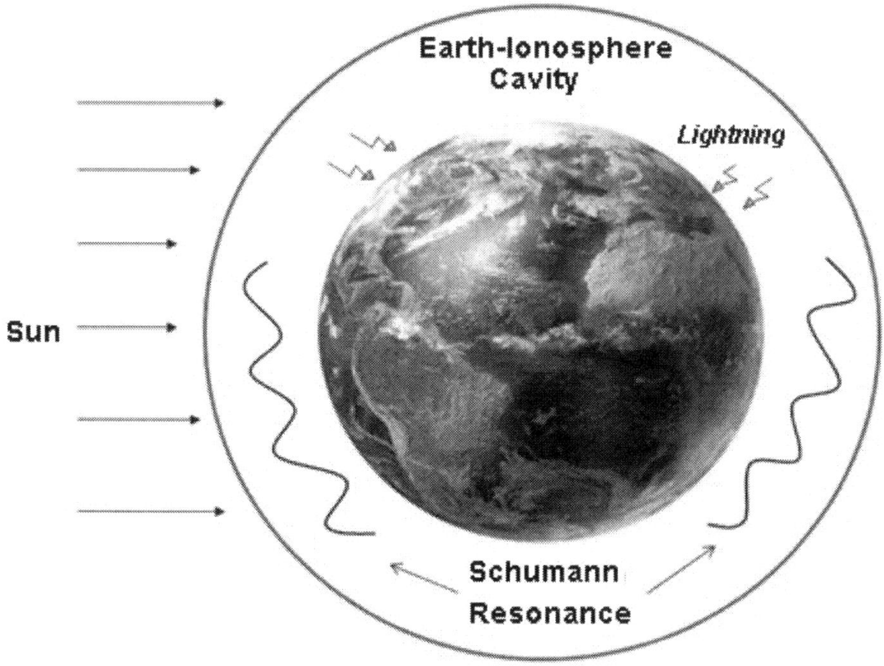

This energy, circling as a wave between the ionosphere and the earth, bumps into itself amplifying frequencies and turning them into resonant waves. The discovery of these resonant waves was made in 1952 by W.O. Schumann, a German physicist, hence where the Schumann resonance gets its name.

In simpler terms, we don't live on the earth, we live inside it. We live in a cavity of sorts. This cavity is created by the connection of the surface of the earth to the ionosphere that surrounds our planet.

Everything within that area, namely energies and frequencies, influence the earth's inhabitants.

Mother Earth's Natural Energies

Although the frequency can spike up or down, the Schumann Resonance primarily levels off at this same measurement...until recently. Lately, frequencies have been lingering around 8.5 Hz, and even as high as 16 Hz.

Even at a stable measurement of 7.83 Hz, the Schumann Resonance is thought to have a great effect on humans and animals. We can guess that these spikes in frequency can have an even greater effect.

There are factors that cause the fluctuation of the Schumann resonance. Influencers such as seasonal changes, solar flares, and electronic interference can alter the frequency at any given time.

The recent increase in the average frequency could also be the result of an increase in human activity, maybe even the increase in human brain wave activity.

Schumann Resonance and the Human Mind Studies show that this phenomenon may indeed affect human consciousness.

The recent increase in measurements may not only be a result of an increase in human brain activity or disruption but can also be the cause of altered brain activity.

We already know that increases in electromagnetic frequencies do affect satellites and power grids, so is it possible that we are being influenced as well.

Basically, it's a connection we've yet to fully understand. However, signs do point to this being the case.

It's also been suggested that the Schumann Resonance can also affect melatonin therefore influencing biological functions such as the circadian rhythm of both animals and humans. Not only does melatonin regulate sleeping patterns, but it also regulates blood pressure and reproduction too.

Some of the worst influences could even include cancer or neurological diseases which can lead to death.

It's believed that human consciousness is affected simply because SR frequencies occur in the same range as human brain wave frequencies, precisely where theta and alpha brain waves intersect.

The Tuned Oscillator Example

The Schumann resonance may be better understood when examining matching vibrations. When a system of oscillators is tuned, one oscillator will affect the other.

When one starts to vibrate, the other will eventually vibrate at the same frequency. Now, remember the fact that our brain waves and SR frequencies are in the same range? This may make better sense now.

This creates "entrainment" or "kindling". The word kindling refers to the matching of neurons across the brain creating synchronicity. This is the same effect that successful meditation has on our minds.

We are in a coherent consciousness, vibrating softly at the same level. With all this being said, meditation keeps our coupling with the Schumann resonance or the fluctuating frequency of the earth.

"Ample anthropological evidence shows that humans have intuitively synchronized with the planetary resonance throughout human history and back into the mists of time."
Psychobiologist, Richard Allen Miller

Many cultures implement vibrational techniques in hopes of synchronizing with the frequencies of the Schumann resonance, or the 'heartbeat of mother earth'.

They believe that these frequencies can heal the body and mind as energies connect. Even in the ebb and flow of these energies, high blood pressure is reduced and depression is somehow alleviated.

Some think synchronizing with these energies can lead us to enlightenment or awakening. It's possible that with the ever-increasing frequencies of the Schumann resonance, we could be evolving into higher consciousness.

Our Connected Frequencies

What we know about our conscious connection with the Schuman resonance is complex. While we know we are influenced by the electromagnetic field, we still have so much to learn.

Considering what we know now, evolution could be greatly affected by the circling frequencies of the Schumann Resonance, increasing activities of the brain and possibly healing aspects of our consciousness previously damaged by negative energies. The future will help us understand more about our relationship with our planet, and the frequencies we share.

٢

Printed in Great Britain
by Amazon

34747840R00042